Praise for *The Warrior's Manifesto*

"*The Warrior's Manifesto*—a treatise that uncovers and delineates the complex layers of an individual acting as a guardian who, at some point alone or in force, might have to make the ultimate sacrifice to save lives. If you carry a gun for a living, you know very well that your choices and actions revolve around four integral human components: life, death, freedom, and money. These elements filter and govern your administration of force. Daniel Modell delves deeply into historical accounts of ubiquitous yet quintessential warrior figures emergent within society at every level who prevent evil in its many incarnations from gaining a foothold on civilization. Through a comprehensive breakdown of events, figures, and battles recorded in antiquity, Daniel compels the reader to believe that the warrior spirit is indomitable and thus remains undaunted."

—Robert Dreeben
Twenty-seven-year veteran, NYPD
Contributor, *Black Belt* magazine and
The Police Marksman
Certified instructor, Wing Chun kung fu
and tai chi chuan

"*The Warrior's Manifesto* delves into the warrior's true motives: the what, why, and way, and the philosophy behind them. I believe anyone in law enforcement, military, and other warrior roles can greatly benefit and be inspired by it. An excellent read."

—Matan Gavish
Founder, Krav Maga Academy

"*The Warrior's Manifesto* raises provocative questions and answers them with depth and boldness. The questions and the answers should inspire meaningful debate at a time when it is sorely needed, a time when the idea and the ideals of the warrior are being attacked and undermined from within and without. The defense contained in the pages of the book will do much to restore the

T0153199

understanding of the warrior professions and the spirit that underwrites them as fundamentally important to society."

—Detective Anthony Amoroso
NYC regional director, New York Tactical
Officers Association

"The men and women of law enforcement, military, and security perform their jobs every day with little praise. They are often ridiculed and criticized for a job few would do. They are told how to do their jobs, but the real 'why' of it all is never truly explained. Over the past fourteen years, I have been privileged to train with these men and women. I am always looking for words to motivate and inspire. I try my best to answer the question 'why.' Despite my best efforts, I was never truly able to articulate this. *The Warrior's Manifesto* answers the *why* and shows us the *way*. It is a must read for any rank or level of experience. It inspires and leaves you feeling proud to be part of that small and very special group of people—warriors. I have often used the word *warrior*, never fully understanding its meaning—until now."

—James Schramm
Police officer (retired)
Senior trainer, Armament Systems and Procedures

"In *The Warrior's Manifesto*, Lt. Daniel Modell (ret.) has presented a magnificent treatise on the warrior mind-set. The exquisitely written book uses artfully crafted historical examples to underscore the lessons and observations he presents. Any casual or serious student of history will immediately appreciate the past examples of courage, fortitude, and a warrior's will to fight for his or her highest purpose. These historical warriors include the likes of Spartacus, King Leonidas, William Wallace, Yoni Netanyahu, and others.

"Mr. Modell places each historical figure not just within the context of the figure's contemporary history but of all history, facing down insurmountable odds—with the key ingredient that each fighter knew the odds were such. Anyone who adheres to the necessity of the 'good fight' will take stock and reaffirm heart from this cogent analysis of why men and women stand up and stand to against aggression. Mr. Modell's insights and writing are nonpareil. This compelling book could rightly be characterized as martial studies, history, philosophy, psychology, military and police science, and possibly a host of other designations—which is what makes it all the more fascinating. *The Warrior's Manifesto* belongs in the pantheon of great books about good versus evil. It provides a comprehensive yet succinct example of why warriors fight."

—David Kahn, US chief instructor,
Israeli Krav Maga
Author, *Krav Maga: Professional Tactics*

Warriors aren't just folks who kill people, break things, and blow stuff up. Sure, violence is often part of the job description, but why and how they fight separates warriors who safeguard freedom from villains who wish to take it away. Modell's treatise is a short but insightful read that cuts to the essence of warriorhood. It'll make you think.

—Lawrence Kane,
award-winning author of *Musashi's Dokkodo*

In this short treatise, Daniel Modell succinctly describes the what, why, and way of the warrior. The historical examples provide guidance for all those who choose the path of the warrior. In essence, *The Warrior's Manifesto* lights the way for all who fight against inhumanity, corruption, and misery: the warriors of our society.

—Alain Burrese, J.D.,
former army sniper, 5th dan Hapkido,
author of *Hard-Won Wisdom*
From The School Of Hard Knocks

THE
WARRIOR'S
MANIFESTO

THE
WARRIOR'S
MANIFESTO

Ideals for Those Who Protect and Defend

Daniel Modell

YMAA Publication Center, Inc.
Wolfeboro, NH USA

YMAA Publication Center, Inc.
PO Box 480
Wolfeboro, New Hampshire, 03894
1-800-669-8892 • info@ymaa.com • www.ymaa.com

ISBN: 9781594395987 (print) • ISBN: 9781594395994 (ebook)

Managing Editor T. G. LaFredo
Cover design by Axie Breen
This book typeset in Adobe Garamond Pro
Typesetting by Westchester Publishing Services

10 9 8 7 6 5 4 3 2 1

Publisher's Cataloging in Publication

Names: Modell, Daniel, author.
Title: The warrior's manifesto : ideals for those who protect and defend / Daniel Modell.
Description: Wolfeboro, NH USA : YMAA Publication Center, Inc., [2018]
Identifiers: ISBN: 9781594395987 (print) | 9781594395994 (ebook) |
    LCCN: 2017960338
Subjects: LCSH: Police—Conduct of life. | Peace officers—Conduct of life. |
    Soldiers—Conduct of life. | Self-defense—Moral and ethical aspects. | Combat—
    Moral and ethical aspects. | Discipline—Moral and ethical aspects. | Violence—
    Moral and ethical aspects. | Martial arts—Moral and ethical aspects. | BISAC:
    SPORTS & RECREATION / Martial Arts & Self-Defense. | PHILOSOPHY /
    Ethics & Moral Philosophy. | SOCIAL SCIENCE / Violence in Society.
Classification: LCC: HV7924 .M63 2018 | DDC: 174/.93632—dc23

Printed in Canada

Contents

Foreword

THUCYDIDES IS OFTEN credited with having written, "The Nation that makes a great distinction between its scholars and its warriors will have its thinking done by cowards and its fighting done by fools."

This Athenian general and classical historian of the Peloponnesian War would have had no need for concern, nor need to caution, had he known Lieutenant Danny Modell and *The Warrior's Manifesto*. Danny is that rare combination of scholar and warrior. With degrees in philosophy from two of the nation's preeminent universities (a bachelor's degree from New York University and a master's degree from the University of Texas at Austin) and twenty years of experience with the world's preeminent police force, he is ultimately qualified to write a contemporary warriors' manifesto.

I have had the privilege and honor to work with and help train many selfless individuals who daily protect our nation, communities, property, and health. Having worked with a cross section of gallant guardians, including military command, Navy SEALs, firefighters, paramedics, and local, state, and federal police, it is clear to me that *The Warrior's Manifesto* provides reflection and direction for any and all members of these elite groups who are committed to attaining the warrior ideal.

However, as my professional experience has been predominantly with law enforcement, I want to emphasize the immense value of Danny's work for police officers. This may be a unique time in the history of American law enforcement, and *The Warrior's Manifesto* is the book for this time.

Never has the police officer been more urgently needed but also scrutinized, criticized, and, at times, even reviled. Among the deserved compliments has been the application of the title "warrior" to those in law enforcement, and this has also been among the heated controversies surrounding the field.

Those who criticize the use of the title in the context of policing seem to demonstrate an excessively myopic viewpoint and failure to recognize the purpose, discipline, and values of the warrior ethos. Unfortunately, the related public and political criticism often demoralizes and erodes the faith, confidence, and commitment of the individual officer.

The Warrior's Manifesto is a tour de force. It is truly a foundation for those who believe police officers can be warriors (and should aspire to be so). It should help relieve the contemporary confusion about what the warrior is and why the appellation does apply to the police officer.

The Warrior's Manifesto will do much to clarify and rectify the real issues. It is both an anchor and a rudder for the modern police officer and police command. The work is a synthesis of the traditions of warriorship and contemporary challenges.

Danny is a wordsmith who writes with an engaging passion and challenging quality. You will not be able to lay this book aside until you have read it all and, until then, you will read with great anticipation of Danny's next point and well-turned phrase. His knowledge of history is truly impressive, but even more so is his presentation of it, which reads not like a stuffy rendition of an irrelevant past but like on-point personal knowledge.

This is a work that the veteran officer will find validating and the rookie will find inspiring. This work will confirm what the veteran officer knows and what the rookie needs to know. It is required reading for both. It cannot be read too soon, nor too often, by either.

Michael J. Asken, PhD
Police psychologist, author (with Lieutenant
Colonel Dave Grossman and Loren Christensen)
of *Warrior Mindset: Mental Toughness Skills
for a Nation's Peacekeepers*, and author of
*MindSighting: Mental Toughness Skills for
Police Officers in High Stress Situations*

The Spirit of the Warrior

T HE SPIRIT OF the warrior touches many across time and place. It is not exclusive to those professionals who devote their lives to it. It touches the mother who, with blinding ferocity, protects a child against danger. It touches the young man who blazes like a flame and charges forward when an armed terrorist storms onto the train that carries him. It touches the principal who plants herself, unyielding as granite, between a machete-wielding madman and the kindergarteners that he means to attack. It touches the brave samaritan who along his way sees a thug robbing an old man and does not avert his eyes but chases the thug away. Circumstances call, and the moment finds a warrior. The spirit of the warrior touches many across time and place.

And what of those who meet not *a* moment but *all* moments as warriors, not by force of circumstance but by choice, under solemn oath, as the sum total of their professional being? To explore the meaning of this choice, of this oath, of this sum total of being across all moments will be our theme here—with no slight intended to the brave souls who answer with a will of stone when circumstance calls out.

The spirit of the warrior is not exclusive to those professionals who devote their lives to it. But it does find its most consistent expression in them. This compass will shape our journey in what follows.

Prologue

SOCIETY MAKES A peculiar offer to its citizenry: we have a job, if you want it. Here it is.

You must stand between the predators and the innocents of the world and hold the line with your blood.

Pay is modest—and rendered grudgingly.

You will labor across hours, long and ungodly, that will test the limits of exhaustion and tedium.

Family will suffer your absence. You will miss many meaningful moments.

You will find yourself shipped to places far away, forbidding, forgotten or assigned to patrol streets savaged by violence, poverty, madness. Your presence will not be welcomed.

You will see tragedy, hopelessness, and evil at depths that will rend your soul. You will be expected somehow, some way, to keep yourself whole as you drown in these so that you may confront them again the next day.

You will be called filthy names. In the course of your duties, you will be attacked, targeted, challenged. Some will try to kill you. They may succeed.

The antipathy of the press and the animosity of the public will flank you without end until your final tour of duty. Your every action, every decision, every remark will be the subject of unremitting—and unforgiving—scrutiny.

Politicians will exploit you—for good and ill—and sacrifice you to expediency once the exploitation is done.

Your mistakes, though honest, will never be forgiven—ever.

You will save many, but the one you lose will haunt you until your dying day.

You will form bonds of brotherhood with your comrades, wordless in their abiding depth, forged in the rough bravery that circumstance compels. You will bury many of those brothers.

You will begin each day knowing that you may never see another.

This is the job that society offers its citizenry. Do you want it?

For most, the answer is an obvious one: no. But for a few, the answer is just as obvious: yes.

This is for the few who answer yes.

I.

The What of the Warrior

Fate whispers to the warrior, "You cannot withstand the storm," and the warrior whispers back, "I am the storm."

—UNKNOWN

EVIL HAS EXISTED in all times and in all places; and in all times and places, those willing to meet evil have also existed. This is the warrant for and the essence of the warrior.

A warrior is not defined by insignia, uniforms, or shields; a warrior is not birthed by bow, sword, or gun. Warriors existed before all these things, and where they don or wield them, bestow them their meaning. If insignia, uniforms, or shields made the warrior, the Nazi Schutzstaffel, mass murderers of the defenseless, would be warriors. Spartacus would not be. A warrior is not defined by insignia, uniforms, or shields.

Fighting for country does not define a warrior. If fighting for country defined the warrior, Japanese soldiers of the Axis who conquered the Chinese and hurled infants in the air to catch them on bayonets would be warriors. The forty-seven ronin of Ako would not be. Fighting for country does not define the warrior.

Fighting for deity does not define a warrior. If fighting for a god defined the warrior, soldiers of the Islamic State, who profess to fight for God as they cleave the heads of "unbelievers" in public spectacles while they kneel bound and unable to fight, would be warriors. Colonel Ethan Allen would not be. Fighting for deity does not define the warrior.

Is it war, then, that makes the warrior?

War has always been a complex affair spanning organization, logistics, and strategy. Staff tends camp, cooks prepare food, engineers design machinery, scribes draft orders. The cook, the engineer, and the administrator may be brave men. Certainly, they are part of the war effort. But as cooks, engineers, and administrators, they are no warriors (though they may be cooks, engineers, administrators, *and* warriors).

Does fighting in a war, then, make the warrior?

From the massive armies of ancient Persia and China to the trimmer forces of France and England centuries later, history finds militaries composed largely of conscripts and slaves compelled to fight at the point of a spear or the muzzle of a gun in an endless procession of predation to extend the imperium of tyrants. Many of those so compelled were brave and skilled fighters, but, had they a choice, they would have elected a different path for themselves. Some embraced their fate. Some volunteered to test their mettle or defend what they believed. They may have been warriors. But those forced to fight in the schemes of tyrants are not warriors. They do not fight by choice for a cause embraced as just.

The long history of warfare, moreover, often stumbles into malignancy unconnected to battle proper. Perhaps the crudeness of conscription feeds the malignancy. In any event, defeating an enemy often meant (and, sadly, means still) raping, pillaging, and plundering. Brutalizing a defeated village is thuggery. Those who do it may be fighters in a war. But fighters, brawlers, and brutes are not warriors. Fighting in a war does not make a warrior.

The warrior existed before any army; the warrior existed before any police; the warrior existed before any shield, sword, or gun; the warrior existed before rank, before hierarchy, before divisions, before units. The warrior exists still above all these things—though he may exist in them too. War needs warriors. Warriors do not need war. Ask any cop.

The trendy cant braying about the "ethical warrior" is therefore a redundancy. It confuses the warrior with one who fights in a war. Nobility was always the pride and mark of the warrior. The soldier, the cop, the freedom fighter must earn the name. It is not bestowed by status or appointment.

History illuminates the theme.

By 73 BCE, the empire of Rome spanned the known world. Its military and cultural power was immense.

Rome was everywhere. To challenge it was madness. One man defied its peerless might. His true name remains a mystery. He kept it for himself. History calls him Spartacus.

Of Thrace and free by birth, "he served as soldier among Romans, after captive and sold as gladiator."[1]

Spartacus was enslaved by the Romans and pressed into death-reeking arenas for the amusement of elites who elevated themselves above others. The elites could do what they would with lesser peoples. They were Romans.

For Spartacus, life as a slave began in the ludus of Lentulus Batiatus at Capua. Existence was harsh in the ludus. To prepare for combat whose end was death to amuse spectators often meant death along the way.

Spartacus yearned for the freedom into which he was born, the freedom wrested from him by a Roman sword. As a skilled strategist burning with life, he hungered for an opportunity to shatter chains. When it tapped, Spartacus seized the day and slashed through his masters to the world beyond their cages. Other gladiators joined. They fought as warriors would, with whatever they could find: kitchen implements, training tools, bare hands. *"Furor arma ministrat"*[2]—rage finds its weapons. Some imagine him rallying his fellow gladiators with these words:

> If ye are beasts, then stand here like fat oxen, waiting for the butcher's knife! If ye are men, follow me! Strike down yon guard, gain the

mountain passes, and there do bloody work, as did your sires at old Thermopylæ! Is Sparta dead? Is the old Grecian spirit frozen in your veins, that you do crouch and cower like a belabored hound beneath his master's lash? O comrades! warriors! Thracians! if we must fight, let us fight for ourselves! If we must slaughter, let us slaughter our oppressors! If we must die, let it be under the clear sky, by the bright waters, in noble, honorable battle![3]

Slaves overthrew slave masters. Spartacus prevailed.

Rome sent Praetor Gaius Claudius Glaber to quell the rebellion. He pinned them on Mount Vesuvius and pursued victory by attrition. But Spartacus was a bold and unorthodox tactical thinker. He scaled down a side of the mountain along plaited vines with a small group of about seventy comrades, outflanked the Romans, and attacked from behind, dispatching the much larger Roman militia, including Glaber, to its end.[4]

Slaves throughout the empire allowed the hope of a once silent word to touch their lips: freedom. They flocked to join Spartacus in thousands. He made an army of them.

Spartacus outwitted, outmaneuvered, and routed legions under command of Publius Varinius. Varinius surrounded the encampment of the rebels. Spartacus posted stakes at regular intervals around its periphery. To the stakes he affixed corpses decked in soldiers' garb, nailing weapons to their hands as he lit fires throughout the camp. The impression from a distance was that of a bustling and well-garrisoned space. Varinius, thus deceived, delayed attack.[5] In the meantime, Spartacus slipped the camp with his army by night, wheeling on the duped Varinius from a better position and destroying his legions.

The Romans clung to the orthodoxy that they were unassailable, that the slave rebellion was but a nuisance. Rome continued to underestimate the will and determination of the rebels—and the leadership and savvy of Spartacus. Its haughtiness was paid in blood. Spartacus defeated legions commanded by Lentulus and Gellius in turn. Each triumph shattered the prevailing dogma that Rome was ineluctable master of the world. Here was a ragtag clutch of disorganized slaves, largely untrained, thought inferior by birth but trim in heart and sharp in will, defying the mightiest power of the day, fighting finally for themselves rather than for the pleasure of others. Other slaves saw it. Rome shuddered in due course.

Finally, when Spartacus choked Rome with its illusions and showed that greatness is not a function of place or birth or class or position, the Senate hurled the full might of Rome against him. Marcus Licinius Crassus, rich, ambitious, and cruel, undertook command of eight battle-hardened legions to defeat the rebellion. To turn in battle under his command meant death. The weight of resources, numbers, and organization was crushing.

Spartacus shifted tactics. Small raids marked by speed and savagery harried Crassus but could not defeat him. Patiently, methodically, Crassus at length maneuvered the rebels into pitched battle and succeeded where others had failed. He defeated the rebels in a desperate and brutal last stand. A strategic thinker as incisive as Spartacus knew its denouement. Finally, he had no delusions about the end of what he started. Rome was, after all, Rome. He might have fled. But where to run when Rome was everywhere? So, he fought.

Though killed on the battlefield, Rome never claimed his body. His men, the men he led, the men who bled with him, the men who breathed but briefly the free air with him, would not yield his body to the abuse of Roman cruelty. He disappeared as he had appeared—in nameless mystery.

Some academics debate his motives and question whether he opposed slavery. This is theorizing among clouds. Spartacus did not, it is true, publish position papers. He was a warrior and otherwise occupied. In any case, outside ivory towers, actions speak. Spartacus fought for his own freedom against those who enslaved him. He fought for the freedom of his brothers in the ludus against those who enslaved them. He fought with seventy thousand slaves who flocked to him against their oppressors. Among warriors, there is no debate. He fought for freedom. And when the fell clutch of circumstance exacted his fall, he fought as a free man against tyranny, the terms of death his own, an equal adversary on the battlefield. *This* was his message: in battle, the pretension of status counts for nothing. Where the final arbiter is blood, skill, and will, the "inferior" Thracian was the equal of the "superior" Roman, whatever the outcome. This was a warrior, his final battle fought in the teeth of defeat to seize deeper victory, for the warrior does not *always* fight to prevail in particular battles. Sometimes the warrior fights for a broader principle, for a future yet unwritten, to reshape thinking, to change the world. He at times fights just to show that it is possible. The unchallenged dogma of the day proclaimed that Rome was and would always be unquestioned ruler of the world. Submission and tribute were the lot of the remainder. Spartacus defied dogma, questioning the unquestioned. History scarcely remembers Crassus, still less Glaber, and less still Batiatus—except as footnotes to the warrior whose true name remains a mystery. Who won the war, then?

Spartacus did not fight under the banner of any nation. He did not sport fine uniforms. He did not fight for the gods. His tactics were heterodox. His army defied traditional structure. He fought, but not for mere brawling. He wished to be free. This, then, is a warrior: one who takes up arms by choice for an ideal, deeply embraced, suppressed or threatened by violence.

This is the what of the warrior.

II.

The Why of the Warrior

We bow down before no man.

    —Spartan heralds to Xerxes at Susa,
    HERODOTUS, *Histories*, 7.136

Whatsoever therefore is consequent to a time or war where every man is enemy to every man, the same is consequent to the time wherein men live without other security than what their own strength and their own invention shall furnish them withal. In such condition there is no place for industry, because the fruit thereof is uncertain, and consequently no culture of the earth, no navigation nor use of the commodities that may be imported by sea, no commodious building, no instruments of moving and removing such things as require much force, no knowledge of the face of the earth; no account of time, no arts, no letters, no society, and, which is worst of all, continual fear and danger of violent death, and the life of man solitary, poor, nasty, brutish, and short.

—THOMAS HOBBES, *Leviathan*, chapter 13

S O, HOBBES. SECURITY from the unremitting peril of "the state of nature" demands society (under monarchy, if we follow Hobbes). There is *something* to this. The enormous time and effort needed to secure basic necessities for subsistence alone in the state of nature is withering. To hunt and gather sustenance, to weave clothing as protection against the elements, to cobble rudimentary shelter from raw material, to manage injuries in the absence of organized medicine, to defend against predation, to maintain fire, and to find water in an unending battle to survive the harshness of nature—which *gives* nothing—is a grueling sentence of stifling sameness unfolding across the tedium of years—and not many of them, as archaeology and anthropology tell the tale. Art, culture, travel, leisure, sport, education, even light, as the sun dims, find no home in the endless, daily drudgery demanded by subsistence. Life in a state of nature is indeed "solitary, poor, nasty, brutish, and short."

That granted, society as such offers no relief from the bleak scape of Hobbes's canvas. Life in the Soviet Gulag or the killing fields of Cambodia is quite as solitary, poor, nasty, brutish, and short. Life for the starving peasant of North Korea groveling before images of the supreme leader while seeking to wrest another day on this earth or for the terrorized wretch navigating the ceaseless factional strife of the Congo is solitary, poor, nasty, brutish, and short. The agglomeration of people under some form of organization as such carries no great value. To be murdered by a thieving rival or stalked by a fanged predator in a state of nature is no worse than to be subject to the more efficient mass slaughter or psychological rape operating under societies yoked by tyranny. Perhaps between the two, if one must choose, the state of nature is preferable, for at least in nature the individual is free—however limited in the range of his possible achievements by external surroundings. Under organized tyranny, freedom is unknown and life, such as it is, continues or ceases subject to the whims of bureaucrats bathing in power.

Whether society carries any enduring value, whether, therefore, it is worth defending, depends centrally on the principles under which it organizes. Defending the existing order regardless of what that order is and what it represents is no sign of greatness and no mark of the warrior. Some are worth defending. Some are not. China under Mao slaughtered sixty million people. The Moguls slaughtered and subjugated millions of Hindus who had done them no wrong across centuries. To defend tyranny; to fight for the practice of exterminating, enslaving, or imprisoning those unlike you; to believe that an individual is the expendable plaything of the tribe, the volk, the demos, the commonweal, the nation-state, or the autocrat—or, what is worse still, to evade the responsibility of examining the belief—is the bailiwick of the bully, not the warrior. Warriors do not feed the gulag with the innocent.

———•———

THE LIFE of the individual citizen is the fountainhead of political value. Societies that treat it as a black-market commodity, exchanged among thieving political operatives in dark alleys, carry no meaning and merit no defense. Liberty is the political expression of the value of each life. Societies that treat it as the punch line to a dirty joke carry no meaning and merit no defense. In an age of relativism, the point is worth lingering over.

Relativism, the intellectual deluge of the age, drowns all distinctions. For the relativist, nothing is true or false, good or evil, better or worse. All is perspective, the universal an illusion. One man's terrorist is another's freedom fighter. The position is stultifying. In its zeal to scold all judgment, relativism finally drowns itself.

Having dismissed truth as an illusion of perspective, relativism can claim no truth itself. Having dismissed right and wrong as illusions of prejudice, relativism can claim no rectitude itself. Strictly, relativism can only claim its perspective—a perspective that is, by its own logic, neither true in any meaningful sense nor good in any moral sense. Logically, therefore, the relativist must ultimately find himself in the precarious position of having no answer for and no objection to the brute who takes a blade to his throat in the conviction that relativists must die. After all, the brute has his perspective too, neither more nor less valid than any other. When this happens, the relativist must pray that a warrior is near—and does not credit relativism.

Alas, many a warrior has succumbed to the spacious delusions of relativism. The peculiar affliction expresses itself in chic and breezy concessions such as "Each is a warrior from his own perspective" or "We fight for the same thing from different sides—we might otherwise have been brothers." The chic concessions ignore context and obliterate the distinction between right and wrong. To say, "The Nazis had their beliefs and fought for them, the Allies theirs. The Allies won, but that does not mean that they were 'right' in some absolute sense. Both the American soldier and the Nazi soldier were warriors," insults the one and elevates the other. *What* you fight for matters. If you fight to preserve freedom against the expansionist brutality of predators who systematically exterminate those unlike them, you can reasonably call yourself a warrior. If you fight for a violent, expansionist ideology that claims the right to exterminate "inferiors" or "unbelievers," you are no warrior. You are a thug. Thugs are not warriors. Terrorists are not freedom fighters.

What *is* worth fighting to protect, then?

In the state of nature, however "solitary, poor, nasty, brutish, and short," the individual seeks no sanction for his life—it is *his* life. The unalterable fact of his existence, requiring his continued action to sustain, is sanction enough. Whether and to what extent he succeeds in sustaining his life is a function of effort, wherewithal, cleverness, and surroundings, but however difficult, however limited in the possible scope of achievement, he disposes his life as he will. His life is its own sanction, its own justification, and its own end.

Consider the alternative: a man's life is not his. If it is not his, then it may be disposed as another decides. Once the premise is conceded, no principled objection to the conclusion is possible. The position cheats reality by thumbing its nose at the evident truth that the individual bears a unique relation to himself—he, and he alone, is master of his person. Another may not own him in the same way and for the same reason that another may not digest his food, suffer his illness, or relive his memories. Those who seek mastery over others deny this truth and seek to substitute their own ends as prerogatives over others who then function as mere means to those ends. But truth sneaks past the denial as the would-be master self-contradictorily insists that *he* not be treated or seen as a mere means to the ends of others. Regrettably, the notion that some men are to be forced to serve as means to the ends of other men, that the life of each is not his own, is a common theme of history and its plot predictable: atrocity and blood. That the individual life is a derivative value, if a value at all, determined by submissive relation to the tribe, the monarch, the tyrant, the class, the race, the volk, the state; that the individual is a mere cell of the body politic, a plaything of the commonweal, which looms menacingly over all as self-appointed sibyls wield it at their whim, is at the root of much mischief in human history. And why not? Under this malignant creed, the Stasi have every right and every duty to crash down doors and toss those deemed "enemies" into reeducation camps or cells or gallows for speaking their minds. Their minds are not, after all, really theirs. They belong to something "higher," beyond good and evil, the public, the proletariat, the aristocracy. The net result is that history is bathed in the blood of those deemed "enemies of the state," "inferiors," "apostates," "untouchables." If a man's life is not his, someone will always emerge and claim the right to dispose it to some "greater" cause, and between those who arrogate to themselves the privilege to dispose of life and those who cling desperately to life, conflict and death must come. It is a reductio ad absurdum in practice. The world can do without it.

How do we preserve the fact that a man's life is inviolably *his* in a social context? *This* is the problem of society.

The answer, in a word, is freedom. Freedom marks the difference between civilization and organized savagery.

I understand that the concept of "freedom" has stumbled through history. The concept developed over time, imperfectly, tripping along as it struggled to find consistent expression as the legacy of all by right, in the teeth of class, birth, affiliation, or geography. But only by groping to understand the principle of freedom and the moral apparatus that it carries can we criticize and reject entrenched institutions, eons old—slavery, subjugation, aristocracy, caste—that have dogged and plagued societies in all times and in all places. In the absence of freedom as an ideal, none of these evils can be opposed as a matter of principle. Slavery is not wrong if freedom is not right.

The warrior is the guardian of civilization, the champion of the aspiration, however halting, that every man is free to choose his path, that no man may set himself above others because of name, power, connections, geography, biology, ancestry, titles, or genealogy from some supposed pantheon. As a corollary, the warrior is an enemy of organized savagery and systemic oppression.

The etymological roots of "society" mean "alliance." The roots enlighten. The will to alliance is more rational and more positive than Hobbes's picture suggests. It is not merely about escaping the peril of nature and avoiding a war of "all against all." Alliance carries enormous advantages. Where the fundamental principle of organization is mutually beneficial interaction under freedom, where each man's life is his, alliances among men in the form of societies birth powerful advantages: enhanced security, burgeoning knowledge, explosive innovation, and self-actualization through division of labor.

When men organize into mutually beneficial alliances and establish institutions to support their administration, they must delegate the right to use force at their whim to an objective agent. Force, in short, must be brought under principled control and strict limits, for force and freedom are opposites. If each were to decide at whim how best to defend against foreign aggressors, how best to apprehend and punish the criminal, and how best to resolve disputes in which he himself is involved, madness and disorganization would follow. Suppose, for example, that two men disagree about where one's property line ends and the other's begins. Each party personally involved in the disagreement would stand as judge and jury for his own case and, invariably, may be counted on to take his own side. With each cemented in the "rightness" of his claim, attack and revenge, arbitrarily administered, are the only avenues of resolution. This enshrines the blood feud of the Hatfields and the McCoys as the idol of human interaction. Finally, whoever is stronger, or whoever assembles the bigger gang, will "win." "Might makes right" becomes the organizing principle of a disintegrating society. Civilization cannot abide under it.

Objective principles of evidence, apprehension, and arbitration, under a framework of explicit laws applicable to all equally, must govern if the incomparable benefits of civilized society are to be maintained. In a civilized society, men must delegate their right to use force against others.

They *delegate* the right. They do not *abdicate* the right. If a man is attacked and the agent to whom the right of force is delegated (that is, in essence, the profession of the warrior) is absent, as often enough happens, the man must of course defend himself with everything he has— and be prepared to explain why. Every man retains the right to defend himself where circumstance compels it. But the special skill of suppressing the initiation of violence by way of retaliatory force in the service of justice is the peculiar province and role of the warrior in society—a role strictly defined and limited to this. To protect against initiated violence from foreign threats requires a skilled military. To protect against initiated violence from domestic threats requires skilled police. To adjudicate legitimate disputes between citizens so that they do not devolve into violence and revenge requires skilled judges, the decisions of whom must be enforceable. Preserving freedom means protecting against the initiation of force. This is the unique role of the warrior.

History illustrates the themes.

By the time Xerxes, king of kings, assumed rule in 486 BCE, the hungry conquests of Persia spanned three continents. Its empire was a tightly controlled network of vassal states radiating from an unquestioned overlord at its center. Xerxes conceived himself a ruler by divine right and, thus touched by divinity, thought to bring the remainder of the known world under heel. Greece was an alluring morsel.

Greece, by contrast, was a bustling, rebellious, free-thinking, and loose network of independent city-states, disposed to spar one with the other, virtually without unity save for language and rough respect for a nascent sense of freedom. Each city-state valued its independence and boasted its own peculiar character. When Xerxes threatened to swallow Hellas, an uneasy alliance of Greeks chose defiance.

Greece had introduced Darius, father of Xerxes, to the difficulties of wresting independence from the defiant breasts of those who valued it at Marathon some years earlier as he sought its subjugation. The lesson did not take. Xerxes pursued the conquest that his father failed to achieve. Divinity brooks no defiance. All would pay tribute by token of earth and water. The Greeks, or some of them, were yet of no tributary mood.

Xerxes meant to escape his father's failure. Over several years he amassed an enormous army conscripted from the breadth of his empire, the living mass pulsating under the stern lash of its captains. Supplies abounded. Oracles assured victory.

Sparta, steeped in the art of combat, was among the defiant allies. When once asked what he knew, a Spartan replied, "how to live free."[6] This is the spirit over which Xerxes sought dominion. The spirit would not yield.

A confederation of allies composed of Corinthians and Mycenaeans, Thespians and Thebans, Locrians and Phocians joined under command of Leonidas, who swore to prove that the "invader was not a god but a man."[7]

In the coming battle, an oracle foretold that either Sparta must fall or a king must die. For Leonidas, king of Sparta, the choice was hardly worth pondering. Sparta would not fall.

Leonidas assembled a group of three hundred of his finest warriors to lead the Greek allies and oppose the immense Persian army under Xerxes. At Thermopylae, Leonidas assembled his men at a narrow pass, under the tactical principle of "not how many but where,"[8] to minimize the strategic advantage of swollen Persian numbers. "Leonidas," someone asked on the way, "are you here to take such a hazardous risk with so few against so many?" In answer, Leonidas said, "If you think that I rely on numbers, then the whole of Greece is not enough for it is but a fraction of their number; but if it is on men's valor that I rely, this will do."[9]

Xerxes, puffed up in numbers and conceit, sent a blunt and pointed demand to Leonidas: "Hand over your arms." In laconic defiance, Leonidas answered, "Come and get them."[10]

Xerxes postured with his bloated army for four days, expecting the Greeks to run at the sight of an unending sea of Persian arms. Instead, the Spartans exercised and combed their hair in preparation for battle—or death. On the fifth day, Xerxes, enraged at length by their impudence at refusing to surrender, sent a wave of his Medes. They charged headlong at the Greeks in vast numbers, but the narrow pass nullified the advantage of number and the Greeks shredded them. Herodotus summarized the message of the first engagement: "In this way it became clear to all, and especially the king, that though he had many combatants, he had but very few warriors."[11] The Greek allies held the pass.

After the Medes had been defeated, Xerxes sent his elite troops, the Immortals, under Hydarnes. They fared no better. They, too, were cut down by Spartan spears in the narrow pass. The Spartans would, at times, wheel about and run as if fleeing, the Immortals in hungry pursuit. The Spartans would then turn suddenly and reform, decimating the Immortals. At length, the Persian army withdrew to its quarters.

The second day of battle saw the Persians again routed in the narrow pass. A contest of arms alone would not defeat Leonidas. Some other stratagem would have to do the work that pitched battle could not.

Ephialtes, seeking riches from Xerxes, betrayed the Greeks by revealing to the king a pathway across the mountain to Thermopylae—a pathway that would allow the Persians to flank the Greek allies. Beginning at the Asopus, Ephialtes steered a detachment under command of Hydarnes along the winding Anopaea, ending, finally, at the city of Alpenus, where, nearby, the Greek allies lay.

Scouts reported that the Persians had discovered the pathway. Leonidas dismissed most of the Greek allied troops but remained with his Spartans, refusing to yield the pass. He understood that yielding would represent dishonor, for the Spartans were chosen specifically to defy the Persian army. He remembered, too, the oracle.

> O ye men who dwell in the streets of broad Lacedaemon!
> Either your glorious town shall be sacked by the children of
>   Perseus,
> Or, in exchange, must all through the whole Laconian country
> Mourn for the loss of a king, descendant of great Heracles.[12]

Sparta—his Sparta, and in it his wife, his children, his warriors—must fall or a king must die. A king must die. Sparta was his heart and his will.

Resolved to their fate and mad with valor of a doom ordained, the Spartans unleashed fury against the Persians, heedless of consequence, for consequence lives in the future, and the three hundred had none. For them, existence resolved itself into a single remaining moment stretching across a strained and desperate present made of will and guts and blood, beyond which there was nothing. They fought, maniacs, a wild current of uncontrolled energy, thrusting spears forward, again and again, under the cramped mass of unending bodies driven toward them by the lash. When their spears shattered at length against a thousand Persian bones, they seized their swords and fought on. When their swords broke under the strain of stabbing flesh, with fists and teeth they fought on. Even doomed, a Spartan is yet a Spartan. Hand to hand, they would not yield, and the Persians could not prevail. Finally, surrounded by archers, a flurry of Persian arrows felled the last of the three hundred, defending the lifeless body of their leader, Leonidas, howling defiance to the end. The Persians won, if you insist.

The victory was short lived. The story of the three hundred excited a nascent sense of unity among the fractious Greek city-states. Soon after Thermopylae, the Athenian navy destroyed the Persians at Salamis. Without ships to supply troops on land, the Persians slowly fell to ruin. At Plataea, with the largest hoplite army yet assembled across Hellas, from many city-states once enemies, the Greeks defeated the Persians and rid their lands of the affectation of tyrants touched by divinity and born to rule over submissive vassals.

Greek warriors fought to preserve freedom and independence, imperfect as they then were, against the pretensions of tyranny; they fought for life as they wished it against the predations of those who would dispose it.

This is the why of the warrior.

III.

The Way of the Warrior

Push off, and sitting well in order smite
The sounding furrows; for my purpose holds
To sail beyond the sunset, and the baths
Of all the western stars, until I die.
It may be that the gulfs will wash us down:
It may be we shall touch the Happy Isles,
And see the great Achilles, whom we knew.
Tho' much is taken, much abides; and tho'
We are not now that strength which in old days
Moved earth and heaven, that which we are, we are;
One equal temper of heroic hearts,
Made weak by time and fate, but strong in will
To strive, to seek, to find, and not to yield.

—ALFRED, LORD TENNYSON, "Ulysses"

IN THE WITCHING hours of night, after a softball game with friends, police officer Stacey Lim was returning home. As she parked, a vehicle carrying five members of a local gang crept behind her. A young man emerged from the vehicle. He meant to murder her and to steal her car. He wanted to prove himself to fellow gang members. Officer Lim stepped out of her vehicle and turned into the looming barrel of a gun. The gang member pulled the trigger, propelling a bullet through the barrel amid the white explosion of muzzle flash and clean through Officer Lim's chest. The bullet ripped through the base of her heart, shattered her spleen, and tore across her diaphragm, liver, and intestines. The blunt impact staggered her. The pain was searing hot. Her fleeting, barely conscious thought was a battle cry: "No time for pain." Get to work. She raised her gun and returned fire. The

gang member fell to the ground. She used the rear of
her vehicle as cover and leaned out to survey the scene.
The gang member was prone, gun still in hand. He fired
at her five more times, missing. She in turn fired three
more times, each one a hit. The remaining gang members
fled—courageous lot, they were. Stacey Lim crawled
toward her door. Her roommate emerged and called
for help.

Blood spilled from Officer Lim. A hundred pints
were filtered back into her as doctors clutched on to her
ebbing life. Her heart stopped. Her body buckled. Having
done all that they could, doctors reckoned it was over,
and said so.

Stacey Lim gave no damn what the doctors said. The
bullet that struck her heart should have killed her. Any
conventional medical assessment necessitated the conclusion. But hers was not just any heart. Hers was the heart
of a warrior, roaring defiance: "There was something
inside me that knew I wasn't going to die." That something inside defied augury; that something inside burned
and raged; that something inside would not yield the
light. That something inside was Stacey Lim's answer to
skulking Death.

Defiance in the teeth of adversity is the central virtue
of the warrior.

Here is the central riddle of the warrior: In answering
the violence of the thug with violence, does not the
warrior merely perpetuate a cycle, adopt, as it were, his

appointed posture in a dance, stepping according to prescribed movements, warrior and brute each doing his part, slave to the scripted step, each different, perhaps, but each no more and no less a dancer than the other?

It is a fair challenge. Here is the answer.

In itself, violence is neither good nor bad. It is a fact, amply asserted by nature, neither more nor less lamentable than any other. The cheetah tears out the throat of the antelope and consumes it. The event is violent, certainly. Is it evil? Of course it is not. Is it good? No more than it is evil. The cheetah merits no moral censure. It acts as instinct drives. There is no choice in the matter. "Good" and "bad" begin with deliberate choice in the face of conscious alternatives. They are functions of human action underwritten by a will that is free, unlike that of the cheetah. In human affairs, then, violence may be wielded for good or ill, depending, like all things, on intention and context. It is a tool, a means to an end, and the means and the ends determine whether the tool is good or bad. Initiated force violates and exploits; retaliatory force protects and defends. Initiated force blinds itself to rights; retaliatory force builds itself around them. The former is evil, the latter good. The pedophile visits violence on a child, though the child did no wrong. Anyone who employs violence to stop the pedophile, to protect the child, does a good thing. Note that the violence employed to protect the child is *not* a "necessary evil." A necessary evil is, after all, still an evil. It is *not* evil *in any sense* to protect a child against a pedophile. It is an absolute good. Protecting the innocent who did no wrong against the violence of a predator is good. Any violence directed against the predator can itself be no violation of right, for the predator never had the right to violate the innocent. If a man shoots another and steals his wallet, he violates the person and deprives him of the capacity to choose how best to dispose his person and belongings, though the victim did no wrong. The violence employed by the shooter and thief is evil for that reason. If a police officer shoots the murdering thief before he shoots and steals, his is an act of protection. He maintains the victim's right to his person and belongings. The violence employed by the police officer is in no sense bad. Protecting life and liberty is good.

Defending the good necessitates violence so long as there are those who would initiate violence. Those who insist otherwise betray the good in practice while feigning care for it in theory. To say that nothing is worth fighting for—"fighting" in a strict sense—to say that the proper answer to violence is "to turn the other cheek," or some equivalent, betrays a curious amorality and demands a vicious apathy. We must not indulge in abstraction here. It serves as a sanctuary for evasion. What is your answer to the pedophile who rapes children? The pedophile will not be convinced that what he does is wrong. Indeed, if he were amenable to being convinced, he would not act as he does. In any event, turning the other cheek yields the child to doom. What is your answer to the brute who plunders the weak, who beats and steals and terrorizes? He is immune to reason, or he would not act as he does. What is your answer? Your answer, if you claim that no violence is justified, is a slave to your premise: you must stand by and watch, the oath of passivity from cowards across centuries. Saying that you can fight for something in the absence of determined, practical action against attack is a rank and paltry dodge. The Nazi is impervious to debate; for him, the blood of the Aryan is the ultimate arbiter of right. The Khmer Rouge does not yield to the sit-in; class in their peculiar sense makes right. There is no word known that, once uttered, stops the sword on its path to your neck. Another sword might, though. If you are unwilling to defend what you believe in practice, violently, if necessary, then your belief is empty. It is a nothing. And you stand for nothing. The strict pacifist is, as a matter of principle, ended by the first thug who disagrees with him. Finally, he does not even defend his pacifism. Nor does he "live" it. He dies—save for the protection of the warrior, who provides him the luxury of his abstractions. As a practical matter, so long as predators threaten life, protectors of life must answer with the only thing *known* to stop violence: violence.

This, then, is the posture of the warrior to violence. Violence is his tool; justice is his goal.

Slogging through the bogs of violence requires a soul of cut steel, a capacity, underwritten by a sense of hope that will not yield, to suppress unraveling under circumstances overwhelming in their darkness. But it exacts a toll. Death, pain, and misery seize the senses; they stake homes in stinging tastes and smells and sounds. Sliding bare skinned along blades of fear and incoherence, swimming against currents of adrenaline, skating the jagged edges of chaos, wrestling fatigue, madness, and hatred leave scars. The scars resist healing.

———◆———

THE WARRIOR can be savage, but he cannot be *a* savage. In the pitch of battle, he fights savagely. But he is not savage for the sake of savagery. Once the warrior has achieved his end, say, apprehending and controlling a criminal, he does not then kick the prisoner who surrendered to show off or gratify himself. To do so is to shade into the province of the brute, for the violence is in that case gratuitous. He shows himself a puppy rather than a professional and his actions assert moral parity with thugs. Why, after all, does he pursue the criminal? Because the criminal visits violence on another without reason in defiance of right. If the warrior visits violence on another without reason in defiance of right, he is the same. Likewise, if a military mission is to seize a town for strategic reasons, the warrior must do all that he can to achieve it. Once seized, the warrior does not then rape and plunder the innocent. He does not dash the brains of infants against walls. His charge is to achieve victory.

It is not to prove a point against the defenseless. To the extent that he does, he initiates violence in defiance of right, to violate, not to protect. The warrior transforms into the thing against which he claims to fight.

The warrior respects rights. His role, after all, is to protect them: to secure the conditions for all to fly where their aspirations and talent will take them and to enjoy the fruit of their effort without fear of being terrorized, brutalized, and erased. This is a deeply human enterprise and, as such, should serve to remind the warrior of his own humanity. Injustice excites in him a powerful indignation. Domestically, the warrior for the working day— the cop—thinks and should think richly about how best to meet the ends of justice. Sometimes it may mean an arrest. Sometimes it may mean a citation. Sometimes it may mean interrogation. Sometimes it may mean incarceration. But, just as powerfully, sometimes it may mean a word of caution. Sometimes it may mean continued tending. Sometimes it may mean "a break." Justice is large and subtle and meaningful. This is why it is an ideal toward which healthy societies strive. Justice is not a petty doodad mechanically applied in quantitative metrics across color-coded graphs. Adopting a broad perspective about how best to achieve it respects the nuanced reality revealed in context. It also pays practical dividends. At least some of those warned rather than cited will remember. Remembering, they may offer valuable information upon a time; they may help the warrior in a moment of truth; they may be the doctors who treat the warrior when he is wounded. Beyond that, remaining sensitive to context and how best to serve justice enlarges one's own humanity. Petty violations are, after all, petty. The spectrum of action available in response to them is richer than a stilted bureaucracy may encourage its members to think.

History illustrates the themes.

William Wallace emerged from the mists of the Middle Ages. His origins are little known. Perhaps he had roots in the lesser nobility. What is known is that he was a brilliant strategist, a gifted fighter, and a proud Scot. And he burned at the English yoke.

Scotland was in some turmoil at the end of the thirteenth century. Dubious successions grounded strife and uncertainty. Edward I, king of England, exploited the weakness and marched into Scotland. Edward forced John Baliol, the weak and nominal Scottish king, to abdicate the throne and seized it for himself. He compelled homage from the nobles. Wallace would not brook submission. He chose defiance.

Wallace employed terrain, timing, and speed to nullify the superior resources and numbers of the English. He harried them with lightning raids from forests dense and forbidding.

Legend has it that he loved as he fought—fiercely. Blind Harry describes Wallace stricken at the sight of Marion Braidfute, the woman he would marry: "As waves, impell'd by waves, his mind is tost, / And in the spreading sea of passion lost."[13]

The English could neither catch him nor best him. After an altercation with the English at a festival, Wallace and his men escaped and hid around the grounds of Marion's home. The English pursued him and demanded that she give him over. She delayed the English soldiers long enough for Wallace and his men to slip to safety. Knowing that Wallace had once again outmaneuvered them, William Heselrig, the English sheriff of Clydesdale, took of Wallace what he could. He murdered the woman he loved. Drowning in the love he felt for Marion, Wallace once expressed to her the worry that he would lose his way, that his "soul would mix and lose itself" in hers.[14] He would worry no more about it. She was gone.

Rage and loss boiled his blood. At night, Wallace and his men slipped into town and surrounded the sheriff's residence. Wallace kicked in the door, charged the stairs, and felled Heselrig, who lay cowering in bed, with a single stroke of his broadsword, splitting the sheriff's skull clean through to the collarbone. His men dispatched the remaining English soldiers.

Wallace embarked on ever more ambitious raids. Success swelled his numbers. Each engagement put the lie to the prejudice that the English were invincible.

As the Scots under Wallace grew in number and came to believe that they could shatter the chains of English rule, a pitched battle between the armies of England

and Scotland had to come. Methodically, through patient movement, Wallace manipulated the English to terrain of his choosing. Stirling was the place. It was a critical entry point to the north of Scotland. In 1297, the Battle of Stirling Bridge would meet history. The armies of England and Scotland faced off. The contrast between them could not have been more striking. The Scots were predominantly a volunteer army, the English largely conscripted under a system of levies on each country that Edward had conquered. The Scots were inexperienced in formal concepts of war, the English schooled in military strategy and hardened in battle. The Scots were few, the English many. But what the Scots lacked in experience and numbers, they balanced with heart and backbone. They were sick to death of English tyranny. They longed for a free Scotland. The English military, by contrast, did what Edward bid, many with weariness and resentment.

To engage the Scots, the English had to cross the river Forth. Stirling Bridge provided the means. The bridge was narrow, allowing but a few to cross abreast. Wallace, like Leonidas before him, understood the tactics of "not how many but where." The narrowness of the bridge nullified the advantage of number. But Wallace had to employ that advantage with delicate precision. On the one hand, he had to wait for enough of the English to cross to damage their army. On the other, he could not allow too many to cross or he would himself be overwhelmed. Wallace waited as his men coiled with energy for the battle. Timing was everything. When enough English had crossed and the bridge was teeming with more, he signaled attack. From high ground, the Scots surged forward like springs, howling war cries from depths that only the oppressed know. Speed and ferocity, their way, added advantage. The English were left unbalanced. The Scots secured their side of the bridge and sealed it. The English on the bridge were now crammed together and effectively frozen with nowhere to move. The Scots gave them no outlet on their side and they were crushed together by those pushing forward from the English side. Many leapt or fell from the bridge and drowned to relieve the petrified suffocation that was otherwise their fate where they stood. Now the main Scottish force flew the slopes, spears level, and plunged headlong into the stifling and stalled English mass. No countermeasure was possible. The annihilation was total. The English lost thousands, the Scots few. The English army thereafter fell to chaos. English commanders sounded retreat and fled. The Scots pursued and killed more. Wallace took the day. Soon after, he was declared Guardian of Scotland.

Later that year, Wallace pressed the attack into northern England, a bold strategy all insolence and presumption, as are all challenges to existing orthodoxy. The attack of this lowly Scot against the eminent power of the day excited disbelief—then terror. Its sheer daring delayed effective counterattack by the English. Wallace scoffed at the pretension of Edward's power.

By 1298, the urgency of Wallace's victories—and what they symbolized—impelled Edward to invade Scotland himself. The adversaries met at Falkirk. Edward was resolved to avoid the humiliation that his commanders had suffered under Wallace's brilliant strategic maneuvers. Edward conscripted an enormous army, well provisioned, favored by all the latest military technology. Heavy cavalry stretched as far as the eye could see.

For his part, Wallace employed *schiltroms*, nests of spearmen in close formation working as one to function as an impenetrable barrier against the havoc wrought by charge of cavalry.

True to tradition, the English cavalry charged. The noise of the charge was fearsome. At first sight of the onslaught, Wallace's own cavalry galloped off the field. Some say it was treachery. Treachery or not, strategically, it was devastating.

The schiltroms held against the thunder of English cavalry, the Scots showing steely discipline against the swift advance of hoof and lance. But Edward had contingencies at his disposal. Welsh longbows, precise and deadly, had an effective range far greater than that of traditional archers. Without cavalry to provide effective countermeasure against them, the Welsh longbows could wreak destruction without impediment. And so they did. Against heavy cavalry, the schiltroms held; against the endless hailstorm of arrows, they buckled. That done, English cavalry and infantry took care of the rest. In the chaotic retreat, thousands of Scots were slaughtered.

Wallace escaped. But he no longer had an army, and Scotland, war weary in any case, had lost a champion. Edward reasserted control.

To the Scottish nobles who had joined Wallace and lately fought England, Edward was lenient. He imposed minor sentences for their rebellion, none of them enforced to any significant degree. His leniency boiled into poison for just one man: William Wallace. His obsessive venom for Wallace, long after he was no longer a threat militarily or existentially, is a testament to what Wallace represented: defiance and freedom. To Wallace, Edward was not the fearsome monarch, divinely installed, to be obeyed. He was a man. And as a man, Edward had earned nothing from Wallace. Perhaps Edward grasped, dimly, the truth in it. The truth could not live if Edward was to maintain power. Wallace had to be destroyed.

Wallace escaped and roamed Europe, rallying other nations to support the Scottish cause as best he could. When he returned to Scotland at length, he renewed his campaign against English rule. He fought again from the forests in raids that flashed and faded like lightning.

In 1305, hoping to parlay with Robert the Bruce, who had sent word for a meeting in Glasgow, Wallace removed to the town and waited. Meanwhile, Sir John de Menteith, a former ally of Wallace who was godfather to his sons, had been enlisted to betray his old friend. Menteith had a history of turning as the winds of fortune blew and, seeing Edward in his ascendency, agreed to capture Wallace in exchange for some lands and position. Menteith surrounded the lodging in which Wallace and his page slept. A bribe ensured that their arms were taken as they slumbered. A throng of Menteith's men ambushed Wallace and a dozen hands were on him as the fog of dreams lifted. What does one do in an ambush? Attack. Wallace fought bare handed with mad rage. He broke the back of one attacker and smashed the skull of another. All rushed him at once, but even together they could not budge him. He would kill them all or die himself, but he would not yield. Then he heard the voice of his old friend, John de Menteith, calling out, promising safety under his protection at Dumbarton Castle. Wallace still trusted Menteith and so consented to be bound. When he emerged from his lodging and saw that his page had been executed, the taste of bitter treachery stung his tongue. William Wallace was now prisoner of King Edward of England.

Edward, dominant monarch of the day, had been bested by this "brigand," a man essentially without land or title, more than once. His vindictiveness at the slights—and what they represented—was unyielding. At trial, a show with the conclusion settled long before Wallace was captive, without even examination of witnesses, his hope

of justice long dashed, friendless, pained by imprison-
ment and neglect, he still refused to beg for mercy.
Wallace still spat defiance in Edward's face:

> I can not be a traitor, for I owe him no allegiance. He is not my
> Sovereign; he never received my homage; and whilst life is in this
> persecuted body, he never shall receive it. To the other points whereof
> I am accused, I freely confess them all. As Governor of my country
> I have been an enemy to its enemies; I have slain the English; I have
> mortally opposed the English King; I have stormed and taken the
> towns and castles which he unjustly claimed as his own. If I or my
> soldiers have plundered or done injury to the houses or ministers of
> religion, I repent me of my sin; but it is not of Edward of England
> I shall ask pardon.[15]

In a lengthy spectacle, he was hanged, emasculated,
eviscerated, drawn, and quartered. He bore the torments
with abiding fortitude. Perhaps he thought of Marion;
perhaps he dreamed of freedom; perhaps he glimpsed in
his own deeds a future struggling to live, breathing still
even as breath left him. When it was done, his head and
limbs were posted throughout England. The publicity of
it all was a standing threat: further rebellion would meet
the same end.

As tyrants always do, Edward miscalculated. The
manner of Wallace's death breathed immortality into his
butchered limbs. As a martyr, he lived in the Scottish
mind, a symbol of what might be, proof that the most
powerful monarch could be bested by the landless, the
untitled, the brave heart yearning to be free.

In 1314, the Scots answered the threat signaled by the display of Wallace's head and limbs. Robert the Bruce, stirring the "Scots, wha hae wi' Wallace bled,"[16] thundered onto the fields at Bannockburn and crushed the assembled English. Scotland was itself again and William Wallace its enduring emblem.

The warrior is after justice. He uses violence. And he meets adversity with defiance—even to his end.

This is the way of the warrior.

IV.

The Best of the Warrior and the Bane of the Warrior: The Leader and the Bureaucrat

We trained hard, but it seemed that every time we were beginning to form up into teams we would be reorganized. Presumably the plans for our employment were being changed. I was to learn later in life that, perhaps because we are so good at organizing, we tend as a nation to meet any new situation by reorganizing; and a wonderful method it can be for creating the illusion of progress while producing confusion, inefficiency, and demoralization. During our reorganizations, several commanding officers were tried out on us, which added to the discontinuity.

—CHARLTON OGBURN JR., "Merrill's Marauders: The Truth about an Incredible Adventure"

I N JUNE 1918, as World War I raged, momentous
fighting roared near the Marne River in France, at
Belleau Wood. The Germans had recently defeated the
Russians in the east, leaving some fifty divisions free to
fight elsewhere. The German army employed the divisions to launch a series of attacks against the Western
Front. The Germans craved Allied defeat before the
United States could invest its full might. Marines already
deployed were directed to hold their position near Belleau
Wood against German advance.

When German infantry attacked, marines held line
and fire with glacial discipline until their adversaries were
practically beard to beard. Marines then unleashed withering volleys of precision fire, leveling scores of German
troops and driving the remainder to retreat. The retreating

Germans dug a defensive line northward through Belleau Wood.

On June 6, 1918, as part of a phased Allied counter-offensive, marines moved from the west into Belleau Wood toward the entrenched German lines. The nature of the terrain compelled the marines to advance through open wheat fields. The Germans had established nests of machine guns and were spraying the fields with a tornado of bullets. Stepping out was a fearsome prospect. The thudding roar, the acrid smoke, the seamless, swallowing sheet of endless gunfire sapped the will of the marines thus pinned and exhausted by days of withering battle. Gunnery Sergeant Dan Daly of the Seventy-Third Machine Gun Company was among the marines so pinned. Daly was modest in stature but in will unbound. He declined commissions. He thought that medals were nonsense. Yielding made no part of his world. He peered at the men of his unit and, with the fierce yawp of the warrior who knows no surrender, rallied them with this challenge: "Come on, you sons of bitches, do you want to live forever?" He leapt from the foxhole and charged the German lines against the twisted symphony of gunfire. Marines of his unit forgot their exhaustion; they forgot their fear; they followed in a surge of forward motion. The sequel was a nova of fury, among the fiercest fighting of the war, much of it close, intimate, expressed in fist, flesh, and bayonet. The marines suffered enormous casualties—the worst in their history.

But they prevailed. They established a foothold in Belleau Wood. The Germans would never get it back.

Leadership knows no rank. The corollary, not repeated often enough, is that rank is no index of leadership. Daly was a leader. He was no officer.

The rudiments of leadership live within every warrior: self-regulation, self-discipline, and self-possession. Emotions do not rule him. Politics do not rule him. What others may think does not rule him. Orthodoxy does not rule him. Institutions do not rule him. The prospect of power does not rule him, nor does the prospect of fame. He is "captain of his ship," his direction and course determined by skill at the helm, not by the aimless buffeting of the waves or the whimsy of the gale, however these may complicate his journey.

Every warrior, then, leads in his own actions. Whether he is leader to others is largely a function of vision: his capacity to define meaning, mission, and means; the courage to steer that vision to reality; and the passion to inspire others to see their stake in it and come along.

Any organization whose fundamental purpose is to protect and defend must have its warriors. Among the warriors, leaders emerge. Over time, mutations that have little to do with protecting and defending also tend to emerge. As organizations evolve, so, too, does the weight of administration, and if the weight reaches critical mass, propagating itself in a furnace of officialism, the cumulative gravity powered by that weight, by the red tape and the number crunching and the procedural minutiae and the data hoarding, explodes into a black hole of bureaucracy, that bloated monstrosity that consumes identity, humanity, responsibility, and decisiveness alike; mashes them through its reeking digestive tract; and excretes through its bowels process, protocol, and paper in their stead. Guardians of the excretion emerge dutifully: rank seekers, power lusters, functionaries—in a word, bureaucrats. Thus, within the same organization, the warrior and the bureaucrat, the leader and the functionary, may exist side by side, the latter affecting by outward show, at least at cocktail parties, what by right belongs only to the former.

Warriors spend their time confronting evil on crime-ridden streets or in theaters of war. Executive managers, the hungriest bureaucrats, spend their time maneuvering for promotion within an organization. These are fundamentally different endeavors. That both types exist within an organization known as "police" or "military" does not mean that both share some fundamental essence. "Police" and "military" are, finally, just words. What a police officer does, what a soldier does, is what matters. What rank he sports says nothing of moment.

This is why chain of command, while it can be an important thing theoretically, is not very important in practice, executive propaganda aside. For the true leader, it is an issue without substantive meaning. A leader of warriors never frets over injunctions, rules, and hierarchies. These are the tools of the bureaucrat. The leader who *earns* the allegiance of his men through the intersection of courage, character, vision, and loyalty requires nothing else. His men will follow him. Musty manuals are not the ground for their allegiance.

A true leader gives no thought to whether his men will follow him or adhere to his orders. But the functionary does and must. Between the leader and his men there is no space to divide. Shared virtue and purpose bind them. By contrast, the space between the functionary and his subordinates is boundless; he divides it by way of politics, vanity, ambition, distrust, careerism, incompetence, and, invariably, a dearth of meaningful experience. Where the leader sees men, the functionary sees subordinates. Where the leader sees his men for who they are, their strengths and their weaknesses, their courage and their folly, the functionary sees his subordinates through a prism of careerism, vanity, and accolade. The world of the functionary is made up of those who might help him secure status and those who might hinder him in securing status. In short, to the functionary, subordinates are utilitarian objects, organs to support his affectations. They hold no other value to a bureaucratic mentality. Warriors know it. Any such manager, whatever his rank, has good reason to fear that his orders will not be followed. Warriors do not and should not sacrifice good men—themselves or their brothers—to serve the careerism of bad ones.

Conferred status, in itself, is no index of competence, decency, or leadership. In fact, given the development of modern bureaucracies, conferred status rather signals a talent for politics, machinations, and obsequiousness. Too often and all too often, the executive indulges vanity by clawing his way up the hierarchy, flattering those above, exploiting those below, and backstabbing peers that affect the same ambitions. This path to power leaves no moral center, and without one, self-worth has no place to abide. The only thing left to the functionary is a thin sense of validation externally driven by his position within the larger organization. Of necessity, whatever propels him forward in the bureaucracy, he will do. He has nothing else. Morally, he is dirty. Politically, he is shifty. Psychologically, he is a blank. Leaders cannot come from such corrupt stuff, whatever nominal rank may fester from it. The bar- and star-hungry functionary is a silent disease weakening the heart of professions that cannot survive but for heart.

By contrast, the leader's sense of worth is grounded internally by a ceaseless drive to develop the best within him. He understands that discipline and excellence are not achieved by rule and whip. Xerxes discovered this truth as his troops were being cut down in thousands by hundreds. Discipline and excellence in the field are culti-vated through courage and confidence and vision. The leader lives these. He needs no rules beyond them, no insignia, no conferred authority; again, these are the trappings of the bureaucrat. Spartacus was a splendid example of how little they mean.

THE BUREAUCRAT represents a special danger to the warrior. While the warrior knows what to expect from his professed adversary in battle, the warrior does not expect to be attacked, undermined, and exploited—all with oily, simpering expressions of outward concern (when expedient, in any case)—by those who don the same uniform, affect the same oaths, and profess loyalty to the same organization. There is no pretense (as to purpose) in battle. Each will do what he must to prevail. But the warrior does not know and, in the nature of the case, cannot know how to fight anything as abstract as the back-room memoranda, political calculations, seatless envy, and artful scapegoating that are the billowing cloaks of executive predation.

The distinct orientations of those who seek rank and those who confront evil within an organization breed toxicity at the top. The disease is worth exploring; it rots an organization from within. Toxic command kills.

Lieutenant Walter Ulmer offers this description of toxic commanders. Driven by careerism at the expense of subordinates, characterized by dictatorial behavior that shanks organizational unity, they embody a cluster of moral dysfunctions: they rarely take blame or share glory;

they are not toxic all the time, or to all people—that is, their character is marked by serial inconsistency; they are rarely if ever toxic when in the company of superiors—that is, pretense is an imbedded trait; they can be charming when the occasion fits—a characteristic, one hastens to add, shared with serial killers and sociopaths; they often have a coterie of sycophants who reappear on their staffs across assignments; most have been seen as toxic by subordinates since early in their careers; superiors either do not know or pretend not to know, and almost never record, their abuse of subordinates, signaling, it is reasonable to infer, collusion in the practices that propelled the superiors themselves forward.[17] Every warrior recognizes the description. Every warrior knows such "commanders."

Toxic command has real-world consequences. In 2010, as war was still stumbling along in Iraq, some thirty soldiers sought the refuge of suicide within a year. General Pete Bayer asked anthropologist David Matsuda to figure out why. Matsuda found that toxic command was a proximate cause in the suicides.

> Oftentimes platoon leaders will take turns seeing who can smoke this guy the worst; seeing who can dream up the worst torture, seeing who can dream up the worst duties, seeing who can make this guy's life the most miserable. . . .
> When you're ridden mercilessly, there's just no letup, a lot of folks begin to fold. . . . Suicidal behavior can be triggered by . . . toxic command climate.[18]

There are some good men in the upper strata of military and paramilitary organizations. So, the true warrior-leader who has achieved rank need not be defensive about this critique of the rank-seeking bureaucrat. The critique is not aimed at him. But the acknowledgment is a small concession against the standing shame of this dirty and largely silent phenomenon, plaguing professions that should not abide it. Turning a blind eye to those who practice toxic command and lust after power is a deep betrayal of the warrior spirit, and of the warriors who meet the call of adversity with brave purpose. They deserve better. The warrior of rank should lead the campaign of moral censure and social marginalization against the rank seeker whose devotion to bureaucracy unseats his devotion to men. A true leader, whatever his rank, should be repelled by those who affect the mantle of leader by way of faux achievement, political appointment, and outward apparel. Defensiveness in this regard badly—and dangerously—misses the point.

History illustrates what a warrior-leader might and should be.

On October 6, 1973, Egypt and Syria jointly launched a surprise attack against Israel. The Israelis were unprepared and outnumbered. On the Golan Heights, some 180 Israeli tanks squared off against 1,400 Syrian tanks. In the Suez Canal, some five hundred Israeli soldiers were overrun by some eighty thousand Egyptian soldiers sweeping deep into the Sinai Peninsula.

Syrian commandos had slipped into the Golan Heights to capture Israel's headquarters. Israeli commandos responded to defend it but were surprised by the Syrians, who had already established a line and laid down withering automatic fire. Israeli commandos were outnumbered and pinned to tactically inferior ground. They were demoralized and desperate.

The command motto of the Israeli military is at once simple and exacting: follow me. Colonel Jonathan Netanyahu, in charge of the unit pinned by Syrian gunfire, lived the oath wordlessly. Against the storm of bullets, he charged forward calmly, fearlessly, with a few soldiers to his left and right, straight at the Syrians. Watching the vision of their commander moving forward, the rest of the soldiers forgot their desperation. They forgot their terror. They followed. One of his men put it this way: "You see your commander and say: OK, if he is going now, I will join him. . . . He gave us the confidence to get up and join him in battle."[19] It was as if his movement invigorated their limbs and pulled them forward. Though outnumbered, though fighting from tactically disadvantageous ground, though ambushed, the smaller Israeli force routed the Syrian commandos.

They followed where he led because he earned their trust, because his courage served as inspiration, because he believed that they were better than what they believed—and his belief made them believe. This is leadership. Netanyahu never gave a second thought to whether his men would follow him and likely did not care whether they would, a fact no doubt not lost on them. This is, perhaps, why there was no question that they would follow. He was going whether they went or not. The purity of courage that rare, the inspiring sense of forward motion in service of right is, for the warrior, his core, his meaning, his religion. Warriors always have and always will follow it.

Epilogue

THIS, OUR WORLD, can be a sad and tawdry cesspool. It can also be a joyous and blinding light. The warrior fights against inhumanity, corruption, and misery that the light may burn a living fire. Brave the night, warriors; watch over the dreamers; fly to the hopeless; shelter the forgotten. For the good in this world, our world, stand even to the last, a single unmoved will of stone against creeping darkness, armed with the silent oath of all warriors from time immemorial: never yield.

Notes

1. Appian, *Civil Wars*, 1.116.
2. Virgil, *Aeneid*, 1.150.
3. Elijah Kellogg, *Spartacus to the Gladiators at Capua*.
4. Frontinus, *Strategemata*, 1.5.21.
5. Ibid., 1.5.22.
6. Plutarch, "Sayings of Spartans," in *Moralia*, 234 [37].
7. Herodotus, *Histories*, 7.203.
8. Plutarch, "Sayings of Spartans," in *Moralia*, 215 [3].
9. Ibid., 225 [8].
10. Ibid., 225 [11].
11. Herodotus, *Histories*, 7.210.
12. Ibid., 7.220.
13. William Hamilton of Gilbertfield, *Blind Harry's Wallace*, bk. 5.
14. Ibid., bk. 5.
15. Patrick Tytler, *The Lives of Scottish Worthies*, 1.2, "Sir William Wallace."
16. Robert Burns, "Scots Wha Hae."
17. Walter F. Ulmer, "Toxic Leadership: What Are We Talking About?" Army Magazine, June 2012, pp. 47–52.
18. Daniel Zwerdling, "Army Takes On Its Own Toxic Leaders," NPR News Investigations, January 6, 2014.
19. Shai Avital, testimony in *Follow Me*, directed by Jonathan Gruber and Ari Daniel Pinchot, New York City, Crystal City Entertainment, Documentary (2012).

Recommended Reading

The broadest and deepest understanding of a subject comes from plumbing a wealth of sources. In exploring the what, the why, and the way of the warrior, I have endeavored to cast my line wide through philosophy, history, strategy, and practice and reel in what riches I could. For those readers who may wish to think and study further on the themes touched herein, I name some sources that materially shaped this piece. The list is of course incomplete. The book owes debts to so many sources, wise and insightful and challenging, that I could not hope to name them all. But what I note is, I hope, a good start for the curious. Read and think on them with the same unyielding spirit that drives the warrior. What they offer is worth the effort.

Appian (fl. ca. 101–ca. 200 CE), *Roman History*. Though significant portions of this weighty history have been lost through the centuries, it nevertheless serves as a primary source for our knowledge of many key events up to the dissolution of the old Roman republic. The books on the Civil Wars remain substantially complete and offer a brief but meaningful account of the slave rebellion under Spartacus and its end by way of Crassus.

Michael Asken, Dave Grossman, and Loren Christiansen, *Warrior Mindset* (Millstadt, IL: Warrior Science, 2010). A detailed and incisive study of the mechanics of mental toughness, *Warrior Mindset* focuses on the practice of developing effective psychological architecture for managing interpersonal human aggression by surveying the established science and ongoing research behind it.

Marcus Aurelius, *Meditations* (ca. 171–175 CE). Warrior, philosopher, and emperor, Marcus Aurelius composed the *Meditations* to commune with and center his own thoughts. Publication was not his purpose. The writing is simple and penetrating, underwritten by the quiet, internal balance characteristic of the Stoic. The language is unaffected and suggests that his status meant little to him. Leadership lived in his bones. "End for once and all this debate about what a good man should be, and be one." Required reading for those who affect the mantle of leader and warrior.

Jeff Cooper, *Principles of Personal Defense* (Boulder, CO: Paladin, 2006). A ruthlessly brief and brilliant treatise by a battle-hardened marine, the core impulse of the work concerns the development of a ready mind-set for navigating personal combat.

Frontinus, *Strategemata* (ca. 84–96 CE). This ancient Roman general gathered tactical and strategic maneuvers from the history of warfare across classical antiquity into neat, brief, and unadorned anecdotes. Although not always exciting, it is always instructive. Its pages reveal a few of the more spectacular tactical feats managed by Spartacus.

Herodotus, *Histories* (440 BCE). "The Father of History" is our primary source on the Greco-Persian Wars, including the Spartan three hundred and the Battle of Thermopylae. The *Histories* remain a rich mine of detail on war, warriors, monarchs, ideas, and institutions.

Rory Miller, *Meditations on Violence* (Boston: YMAA, 2008). Miller is engaging and provocative in both style and content. The book explores the high-stakes, time-compressed dynamics of real-world violence and questions the application and relevance of traditional martial arts to that context. The insights offered along the way are subtle and powerful. The reader is treated to gripping discussions of violence by type, of violence as an expression of evolution within given contexts, and of violence underwritten and clouded by myth. In the best sense, the book challenges orthodoxy and assumption.

Thomas Paine, *The American Crisis* (1776–1783). Anything by Paine drips with the desperate yearning for freedom and the vibrant energy of revolution so expressive of the Enlightenment in practice. The soaring, combative oratory of the pamphlets that make *The American Crisis* inspired colonists, not least the Continental army soldiers to whom they were read, toward their highest ideals during the Revolution—however dear the cost. Paine articulates in splendid language that which the warrior fights for and against, and more, of course. "These are the times that try men's souls. The summer soldier and the sunshine patriot will, in this crisis, shrink from the service of their country; but he that stands it *now*, deserves the love and thanks of man and woman. Tyranny, like hell, is not easily conquered; yet we have this consolation with us, that the harder the conflict, the more glorious the triumph." Such words transcend age and inspire still.

Plutarch (ca. 45–120 CE), *Moralia*. Of particular interest in this broad-ranging work are the books "Sayings of Kings and Commanders," "Sayings of the Romans," "Sayings of the Spartans," and "Sayings of Spartan Women." Much of how we think about the character and customs of Sparta is rooted in the work of Plutarch.

Sun Tzu (fl. 400–301 BCE), *Art of War*. The value and appeal of the *Art of War* has spanned centuries. It is a network of maxims on the nature of war and warrior, vaulting between practical strategy and philosophical reflection. Oracular in style, it requires some interpretation to glean meaning, but the effort pays.

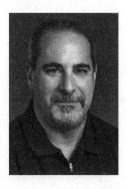

About the Author

D ANIEL MODELL served for twenty years in the New York City Police Department across a range of patrol commands and assignments. Twice promoted during his tenure, he retired as a lieutenant. He was coordinator of the Tactical Training Unit and training coordinator of the Firearms and Tactics Section. He is a certified force science analyst and functioned, during his tenure with the agency and beyond, as an expert in use of force for criminal and civil cases.

Modell is adjunct professor at the State University of New York–FIT, where he developed the curriculum for and teaches "The Art and Practice of Self-Defense."

He is chief executive officer of Ares Tactical and Emergency Management Solutions, which administers self-defense and tactical training seminars to a broad range of institutions.

Modell has published a number of articles, including *The Psychology of the Active Killer, Mythologizing Killers: How Language Distorts Debate and Response, The Roots of the Reactive Posture* and *Case Law and Decision Making.* Daniel Modell resides in Bronx, New York.

BOOKS FROM YMAA

6 HEALING MOVEMENTS
101 REFLECTIONS ON TAI CHI CHUAN
108 INSIGHTS INTO TAI CHI CHUAN
ADVANCING IN TAE KWON DO
ANALYSIS OF SHAOLIN CHIN NA 2ND ED
ANCIENT CHINESE WEAPONS
THE ART AND SCIENCE OF STAFF FIGHTING
ART OF HOJO UNDO
ARTHRITIS RELIEF, 3D ED.
BACK PAIN RELIEF, 2ND ED.
BAGUAZHANG, 2ND ED.
BRAIN FITNESS
CARDIO KICKBOXING ELITE
CHIN NA IN GROUND FIGHTING
CHINESE FAST WRESTLING
CHINESE FITNESS
CHINESE TUI NA MASSAGE
CHOJUN
COMPREHENSIVE APPLICATIONS OF SHAOLIN CHIN NA
CONFLICT COMMUNICATION
CROCODILE AND THE CRANE: A NOVEL
CUTTING SEASON: A XENON PEARL MARTIAL ARTS THRILLER
DEFENSIVE TACTICS
DESHI: A CONNOR BURKE MARTIAL ARTS THRILLER
DIRTY GROUND
DR. WU'S HEAD MASSAGE
DUKKHA HUNGRY GHOSTS
DUKKHA REVERB
DUKKHA, THE SUFFERING: AN EYE FOR AN EYE
DUKKHA UNLOADED
ENZAN: THE FAR MOUNTAIN, A CONNOR BURKE MARTIAL
    ARTS THRILLER
ESSENCE OF SHAOLIN WHITE CRANE
EVEN IF IT KILLS ME
EXPLORING TAI CHI
FACING VIOLENCE
FIGHT BACK
FIGHT LIKE A PHYSICIST
THE FIGHTER'S BODY
FIGHTER'S FACT BOOK
FIGHTER'S FACT BOOK 2
FIGHTING THE PAIN RESISTANT ATTACKER
FIRST DEFENSE
FORCE DECISIONS: A CITIZENS GUIDE
FOX BORROWS THE TIGER'S AWE
INSIDE TAI CHI
KAGE: THE SHADOW, A CONNOR BURKE MARTIAL ARTS
    THRILLER
KARATE SCIENCE
KATA AND THE TRANSMISSION OF KNOWLEDGE
KRAV MAGA PROFESSIONAL TACTICS
KRAV MAGA WEAPON DEFENSES
LITTLE BLACK BOOK OF VIOLENCE
LIUHEBAFA FIVE CHARACTER SECRETS
MARTIAL ARTS ATHLETE
MARTIAL ARTS INSTRUCTION
MARTIAL WAY AND ITS VIRTUES
MASK OF THE KING
MEDITATIONS ON VIOLENCE
MERIDIAN QIGONG EXERCISES
MIND/BODY FITNESS
THE MIND INSIDE TAI CHI
THE MIND INSIDE YANG STYLE TAI CHI CHUAN
MUGAI RYU
NATURAL HEALING WITH QIGONG
NORTHERN SHAOLIN SWORD, 2ND ED.
OKINAWA'S COMPLETE KARATE SYSTEM: ISSHIN RYU
THE PAIN-FREE BACK
PAIN-FREE JOINTS
POWER BODY
PRINCIPLES OF TRADITIONAL CHINESE MEDICINE

THE PROTECTOR ETHIC
QIGONG FOR HEALTH & MARTIAL ARTS 2ND ED.
QIGONG FOR LIVING
QIGONG FOR TREATING COMMON AILMENTS
QIGONG MASSAGE
QIGONG MEDITATION: EMBRYONIC BREATHING
QIGONG MEDITATION: SMALL CIRCULATION
QIGONG, THE SECRET OF YOUTH: DA MO'S CLASSICS
QUIET TEACHER: A XENON PEARL MARTIAL ARTS THRILLER
RAVEN'S WARRIOR
REDEMPTION
ROOT OF CHINESE QIGONG, 2ND ED.
SCALING FORCE
SENSEI: A CONNOR BURKE MARTIAL ARTS THRILLER
SHIHAN TE: THE BUNKAI OF KATA
SHIN GI TAI: KARATE TRAINING FOR BODY, MIND, AND SPIRIT
SIMPLE CHINESE MEDICINE
SIMPLE QIGONG EXERCISES FOR HEALTH, 3RD ED.
SIMPLIFIED TAI CHI CHUAN, 2ND ED.
SIMPLIFIED TAI CHI FOR BEGINNERS
SOLO TRAINING
SOLO TRAINING 2
SUDDEN DAWN: THE EPIC JOURNEY OF BODHIDHARMA
SUMO FOR MIXED MARTIAL ARTS
SUNRISE TAI CHI
SUNSET TAI CHI
SURVIVING ARMED ASSAULTS
TAE KWON DO: THE KOREAN MARTIAL ART
TAEKWONDO BLACK BELT POOMSAE
TAEKWONDO: A PATH TO EXCELLENCE
TAEKWONDO: ANCIENT WISDOM FOR THE MODERN WARRIOR
TAEKWONDO: DEFENSES AGAINST WEAPONS
TAEKWONDO: SPIRIT AND PRACTICE
TAO OF BIOENERGETICS
TAI CHI BALL QIGONG: FOR HEALTH AND MARTIAL ARTS
TAI CHI BALL WORKOUT FOR BEGINNERS
TAI CHI BOOK
TAI CHI CHIN NA: THE SEIZING ART OF TAI CHI CHUAN, 2ND
    ED.
TAI CHI CHUAN CLASSICAL YANG STYLE, 2ND ED.
TAI CHI CHUAN MARTIAL APPLICATIONS
TAI CHI CHUAN MARTIAL POWER, 3RD ED.
TAI CHI CONNECTIONS
TAI CHI DYNAMICS
TAI CHI FOR DEPRESSION
TAI CHI IN 10 WEEKS
TAI CHI QIGONG, 3RD ED.
TAI CHI SECRETS OF THE ANCIENT MASTERS
TAI CHI SECRETS OF THE WU & LI STYLES
TAI CHI SECRETS OF THE WU STYLE
TAI CHI SECRETS OF THE YANG STYLE
TAI CHI SWORD: CLASSICAL YANG STYLE, 2ND ED.
TAI CHI SWORD FOR BEGINNERS
TAI CHI WALKING
TAIJIQUAN THEORY OF DR. YANG, JWING-MING
TENGU: THE MOUNTAIN GOBLIN, A CONNOR BURKE MARTIAL
    ARTS THRILLER
TIMING IN THE FIGHTING ARTS
TRADITIONAL CHINESE HEALTH SECRETS
TRADITIONAL TAEKWONDO
TRAINING FOR SUDDEN VIOLENCE
THE WARRIOR'S MANIFESTO
WAY OF KATA
WAY OF KENDO AND KENJITSU
WAY OF SANCHIN KATA
WAY TO BLACK BELT
WESTERN HERBS FOR MARTIAL ARTISTS
WILD GOOSE QIGONG
WINNING FIGHTS
WOMAN'S QIGONG GUIDE
XINGYIQUAN

DVDS FROM YMAA

more products available from . . .
YMAA Publication Center, Inc. 楊氏東方文化出版中心
1-800-669-8892 • info@ymaa.com • www.ymaa.com